BOILED EGG DIET

I BET YOU NEVER KNEW THIS ABOUT THE

BOILED EGG DIET

DR. J. SIMON

Contents

INTRODUCTION

The Boiled Egg Diet, as its name suggests, is a short-term, high-protein, low-carb diet that heavily emphasizes eating boiled eggs as your primary source of protein. The regimen, which typically lasts for two weeks, promises to promote quick weight loss. However, these diets should be used with caution as they may not offer the proper ratio of nutrients for long-term health.

The main tenet of the boiled egg diet is to stick to a certain list of foods, which includes grapefruit, eggs, lean proteins, and non-starchy vegetables. It usually entails restricting other food groups, such carbohydrates and fats, which creates a calorie deficit and aids in weight loss.

It's critical to realize that while some people may experience rapid weight loss over the two-week period, these diets may not be long-lasting or sufficient in nutrients for overall health. Always seek medical guidance or advise from a certified dietitian before starting any restrictive diet to ensure it is suitable for your specific goals and needs. Remember that long-term health requires sustainable and balanced dietary practices.

CHAPTER ONE

An Overview of the Boiled Egg Diet

The Boiled Egg Diet is a two-week weight-loss plan that is extremely brief. You guessed it: cooking eggs is the central theme. The idea is to create a calorie deficit by limiting fats and carbohydrates and using eggs as the primary source of protein. The diet consists of non-starchy vegetables, lean proteins, and sometimes grapefruit.

Eggs are highlighted because they are low in calories and high in protein, both of which can help with weight loss and fullness. But it's crucial to keep in mind that any diet with a lot of limitations needs to be followed carefully.

Consult a physician or nutritionist to ensure you are receiving the necessary nutrients. While immediate fixes can have an impact, balanced, long-term habits are the key to long-term health.

Basics of the Boiled Egg Diet

Typically, the Boiled Egg Diet involves adhering to a predetermined two-week meal plan. Here are several essentials:

Egg-centric meals consist of cooked eggs as the primary dish. Eating two to three eggs a day, generally for breakfast, may be part of the diet.

Lean proteins: In addition to eggs, lean proteins such as fish, chicken, or tofu can be included to meals. This helps maintain the emphasis on protein and low on carbs.

Non-starchy vegetables: Some of the most often suggested vegetables are broccoli, spinach, and asparagus. They are low in calories and high in essential nutrients.

Restrictions on fats and carbs: Dietary restrictions frequently apply to the amount of fats and carbs that are consumed. It is essential to cut out on bread, pasta, and other high-fat foods.

Grapefruit inclusion: Some diets advise incorporating grapefruit into meals due to its purported ability to increase metabolism.

Portion control: One popular tactic for cutting calories is to limit portions.

It's imperative to stay hydrated and to pay attention to your body. Even though some people may lose weight right away, not everyone should follow such a strict diet. Before making significant dietary changes, one should always consult a healthcare professional. Keep in mind that balance and sustainability are necessary for long-term health.

Dietary Guidelines and Principles

The Boiled Egg Diet often follows a set of guidelines in order to be effective. Here's a general synopsis:

Egg consumption: Cooked eggs are usually the diet's primary source of protein. This is normally for breakfast and might range from two to three eggs per day.

Low carb, high protein: A high-protein diet is recommended to promote fullness and muscle preservation. Carbohydrates are often restricted to create a calorie deficit.

Lean proteins: In addition to eggs, lean protein sources that can be added to meals include fish, tofu, and chicken.

Non-starchy vegetables: Broccoli, spinach, and kale are good choices because of their low calorie count and excellent nutritional value.

Limits on fats and carbohydrates: In general, the diet places restrictions on the amount of fats and carbohydrates that are ingested, so high-fat items like bread and pasta are off limits.

Portion control: It's customary to place a high priority on keeping reasonable portions in order to control overall caloric intake.

Hydration: To stay hydrated and support overall wellbeing, it is usually recommended to consume a lot of water.

Incorporate grapefruit into meals: Some diets advise incorporating grapefruit into meals because of its alleged capacity to boost metabolism.

Remember that while the Boiled Egg Diet could lead to a brief reduction of weight, these kind of rigid routines ought to be used with prudence. Consult a dietitian or other medical professional to be sure it meets your needs and health objectives. Sustainable and well-balanced dietary practices are crucial for long-term health.

Crucial Components of the Diet

Typically, the Boiled Egg Diet includes these several key components:

Eggs: Boiled eggs are the primary source of protein and the major focus of this diet. Many people consume eggs for breakfast, and some diets may require a specific number of eggs per day.

Lean Proteins: In addition to eggs, lean protein sources like chicken, fish, and tofu are used to provide variety and ensure an adequate intake of essential amino acids.

Non-starchy Vegetables: Rich in nutrients and low in calories, these veggies include spinach, asparagus, and broccoli. They contribute fiber to the diet as well.

Restricted Carbohydrates: Carbohydrates, especially refined ones like bread and pasta, are typically restricted in order to create a calorie deficit and help with weight loss.

Reduced Fats: Reducing fats, especially saturated fats, is typically an element of a diet. This contributes to the overall reduction in calories.

Grapefruit: Several Boiled Egg Diet variations include grapefruit because it is believed to speed up metabolism and help with weight loss.

Portion control: Keeping an eye on portion sizes is a well-liked tactic for cutting calories overall.

Remember that while the diet might help you lose weight quickly, you should exercise caution when implementing it. A medical professional or dietitian should be consulted before starting any restrictive diet plan because extreme restriction can deprive the body of essential nutrients.

The Nutritional Worth of Hard-Boiled Eggs

Boiling eggs are a nutritional powerhouse that provide many essential nutrients in a small, portable package. An overview of their nutritional value is provided below:

Protein: Since eggs contain every essential amino acid needed for a number of bodily functions, they are an excellent source of high-quality protein.

Vitamins: Eggs are a good source of B vitamins, including folate, B2 (riboflavin), B5 (pantothenic acid), B6 (pyridoxine), and B12 (cobalamin). They also contain the vitamins A, D, E, and K.

Minerals: Among the minerals that are abundant in eggs are iron, phosphorus, zinc, and selenium. Maintaining general health requires these minerals.

Good Fats: While there is some fat in eggs, it's mostly unsaturated fat, like the heart-healthy omega-3 fatty acids.

One of the best food sources of choline, which is necessary for healthy liver, brain, and metabolism, is eggs.

Yogurt contains the antioxidants lutein and zeaxanthin, which reduce the risk of age-related macular degeneration and enhance eye health.

It's crucial to remember that many elements, such the size of the egg and the preparation technique, might affect the nutritional content. Because boiling keeps the nutritional value of the egg and doesn't add unnecessary fat, it's a healthy way to cook eggs.

Advantages and Demands

The boiled egg diet is frequently linked to a number of assertions and possible advantages, but it's important to view these cautiously. Among the benefits and claims that are frequently highlighted are:

Rapid Weight Loss: Losing weight quickly is one of the main promises. The diet's emphasis on protein and limitations on fats and carbohydrates may cause a calorie deficit that results in weight loss over the short term.

Enhanced Metabolism: Some diets include grapefruit, which is said to increase metabolism and aid in weight loss.

Reduced Calorie Intake and Satiety: High-protein diets, such as the Boiled Egg Diet, may increase feelings of fullness, which may lead to a reduction in total caloric intake.

Nutrient-Dense: Rich in protein, vitamins, and minerals, among other nutrients, eggs contribute to a diet's total intake of nutrients.

Easy Meal Plan: One of the diet's main selling points is its simplicity, which makes it accessible to people who are searching for simple meal plans. It is also known for being easy to follow.

It's important to remember that while some people may lose weight initially when following the Boiled Egg Diet, these claims may not apply to everyone. Furthermore, the restrictive nature of the diet may not be long-term maintainable and may result in dietary deficiencies. Prior to beginning any restrictive diet, always check with a medical expert or a certified dietitian to make sure it is appropriate for your particular health needs. Sustainable and well-balanced dietary practices are essential for long-term health.

CHAPTER TWO

Recipes and Meal Plans

Here is an example meal plan that follows the general guidelines of the Boiled Egg Diet, though exact meal plans and dishes may differ:

First Day:

Two boiled eggs and a grapefruit for breakfast

Lunch would include steamed broccoli and grilled chicken breast.

Dinner is spinach salad on the side and boiled eggs.

Day 2:

Two boiled eggs and one avocado for breakfast

Lunch would be mixed greens and tuna salad.

Supper will be baked fish and asparagus.

Day Three:

Two boiled eggs and a tiny apple for breakfast

Lunch would be a stir-fried tofu or turkey with non-starchy vegetables.

Dinner is kale salad and boiled eggs.

Day Four:

2 cooked eggs and 1/2 cup fruit for breakfast

Lunch would be chicken or shrimp lettuce wraps.

Dinner is roast Brussels sprouts and grilled fish.

Day Five:

Oysters and two boiled eggs for breakfast

Lunch would be cucumber slices and egg salad.

Dinner is vegetarian chili or lean beef.

Always remember to stay hydrated by sipping lots of water all day long. Modify serving sizes according to specific needs and seek the assistance of a nutritionist or healthcare provider for individualized guidance. Although this gives you a rough concept, it is important to make sure the diet is balanced and fulfills your nutritional needs.

Taking Into Account and Precautions

It's crucial to take the following safety measures into account before beginning the Boiled Egg Diet or any other restricted diet:

Nutrient Deficiency: Because the diet is so limited, it may not provide enough of several vital nutrients. To satisfy your body's nutritional demands, make sure you're eating a range of meals.

Sustainability: The Boiled Egg Diet is a transient strategy that could not work in the long run. For long-lasting health, concentrate on creating balanced, long-term dietary habits.

Individual Variability: Everybody has different nutritional needs. What suits one person might not be appropriate for another. For individualized guidance, speak with a nutritionist or other medical practitioner.

Possible negative Effects: Excessive weight loss may cause exhaustion, lightheadedness, and vitamin shortages, among other negative effects. Observe how your body reacts, and if necessary, seek medical assistance.

Heart Health: The high egg content of the diet may cause one to worry about cholesterol intake. Although most people's blood cholesterol is not significantly affected by dietary cholesterol, those who already have cardiac problems should use caution.

Hydration: Make sure you drink enough water, as diets high in protein can make you require more. Throughout the day, water is the greatest beverage for you.

Balanced Exercise: Make frequent exercise a part of your daily schedule. Exercise is essential for general health and goes well with a well-rounded diet.

Consultation with Experts: Speak with a certified dietitian or a healthcare provider before beginning any diet, especially one that is restrictive. Taking into account your objectives and medical history, they can offer tailored guidance.

Recall that balanced and sustainable lifestyle and eating choices are critical to long-term health. If losing weight is your objective, the best way to do it is to combine a nutritious diet with consistent exercise and thoughtful living decisions.

Obstacles and Remarks

Like many restricted diets, the boiled egg diet has its share of drawbacks and critics.

Nutrient Imbalance: The diet's emphasis on a small number of foods may provide an unbalanced intake of vital nutrients, which could result in vitamin and mineral shortages.

Unsustainability: The diet may be difficult to stick to over time due to its restricted nature. Fast cures frequently don't have long-term effects, and going back to one's former eating patterns can cause weight gain.

The diet's heavy emphasis on eggs may give rise to worries over cholesterol consumption. For most people, the effect of dietary cholesterol on blood cholesterol is minimal; nevertheless, individuals who already have cardiac problems should exercise caution.

Possible Side Effects: Excessive weight loss can have unfavorable effects like weariness, lightheadedness, and stomach problems. Extreme calorie restriction may also have an effect on one's general wellbeing and energy levels.

Limited Food Variety: The diet's monotony may make it less pleasurable, which could cause problems with adherence. A varied diet is essential for a balanced and fulfilling intake of nutrients.

Lack of Strong Scientific Evidence: There is insufficient evidence to support the effectiveness and health advantages of the boiled egg diet. The best weight loss strategies are those that are balanced and grounded in science.

Individual Variability: Everybody has different nutritional needs. What suits one person might not be appropriate for another. It is essential to get individualized guidance from medical specialists or nutritionists.

Prioritize Weight Over Health: The diet's emphasis on quick weight loss may take precedence over the value of general health. Sustainable health calls for a multifaceted strategy that takes into account all facets of wellbeing.

Before making big changes to your eating habits, it's important to approach any diet, including the Boiled Egg Diet, cautiously and speak with dietitians or medical professionals. For long-term health, sustainable and well-balanced nutrition strategies are essential.

CHAPTER THREE

Although the Boiled Egg Diet can result in quick weight loss, there are some possible health hazards and warnings related to this rigorous eating schedule:

Nutrient Deficiency: Because the diet isn't rich in a variety of foods that are required to different food groups, it may not contain the full range of nutrients that are needed.

Cholesterol Concerns: Eating a lot of eggs in the diet may lead to consuming more cholesterol. While not everyone is impacted by dietary cholesterol in the same manner, those who already have cardiac problems or high cholesterol should exercise caution.

Digestive Problems: Some people may experience bloating, gas, or constipation as a result of a sudden increase in egg consumption.

Energy Levels: Due to the low calorie content of the diet, you may feel less energetic, tired, and find it harder to stay active.

Concerns about Sustainability: The Boiled Egg Diet is a temporary strategy that might not be viable in the long run. Fast remedies frequently only produce short-term effects, and going back to your old eating patterns can cause you to gain weight.

Possibility of Muscle Loss: The diet's emphasis on rigorous calorie restriction may cause lean muscle mass to be lost, which would alter the composition of the body as a whole.

Impact on Metabolic Rate: Extremely low-calorie diets may cause the metabolism to momentarily slow down while the body adjusts to consuming less calories, which will make it more difficult to sustain weight loss over the long run.

Individual Variability: Everybody has different nutritional needs. What suits one person might not be appropriate for another. Take into account certain medical issues and consult a specialist.

It is imperative to speak with a medical expert or a qualified dietitian prior to beginning any restrictive diet, including the Boiled Egg Diet.

They may offer tailored advice based on your objectives and medical history, making sure that you tackle weight reduction and general well-being in a sustainable and safe way.

Sustainable Approaches and Alternatives

The following strategies should be taken into consideration if you're seeking for more long-term, sustainable alternatives to the boiled egg diet:

A balanced diet

Prioritize eating a diverse and well-balanced diet that consists of a range of fruits, vegetables, whole grains, lean meats, and healthy fats.

To maintain general health, make sure you consume a variety of nutrients from various food sources.

Control of Portion:

To balance calorie intake without unduly reducing food groups, use portion management.

To prevent overindulging, use smaller dishes and pay attention to serving amounts.

Frequent Exercise:

Exercise on a regular basis to improve your general health and control your weight.

Make physical activity a sustainable component of your lifestyle by engaging in activities you enjoy.

Consciously Consuming Food:

Observe your body's signals of hunger and fullness.

Savor your food and eat slowly, letting your body tell you when it's full.

The Focus on Whole Foods:

Give whole, unprocessed foods the upper hand over heavily processed ones.

Select meals that are high in nutrients and contain fiber, vitamins, and minerals.

Drink water to stay hydrated throughout the day.

Water should be your main beverage of choice; limit sugar-filled drinks.

Adaptable Consumption Habits:

Investigate adaptable eating habits that fit your preferences and lifestyle, such as mindful eating or intermittent fasting.

Professional Consultation:

Seek assistance from medical specialists or qualified dietitians, who can offer tailored recommendations based on your unique health requirements and objectives.

Recall that long-term lifestyle adjustments are more important for sustainable weight management than sporadic, restrictive diets. To achieve and sustain total well-being, a holistic strategy incorporating mindful eating, frequent physical activity, and balanced diet is essential.

CONCLUSION

To sum up, the Boiled Egg Diet is a brief, low-calorie eating regimen that prioritizes the consumption of lean proteins, non-starchy vegetables, and boiled eggs in order to promote rapid weight loss. Although this strategy may initially work for some people, there are a number of possible negative effects and health hazards.

The diet's drawbacks, which include dietary shortages, cholesterol problems, and sustainability concerns, cast doubt on the plan's long-term efficacy and effects on general health. The emphasis on quick weight loss could obscure the value of long-term, well-rounded nutritional strategies.

Seek advice from medical specialists or licensed dietitians before beginning any restrictive diet, including the Boiled Egg Diet. They can offer tailored advice that takes into consideration specific health issues and objectives, as well as assist in creating a long-term, viable plan for wellbeing.

In general, more sustainable and successful strategies for reaching and maintaining a healthy weight include selecting a varied, balanced diet, controlling portions, getting regular exercise, and developing mindful eating habits.

THE END